Rheumatoid Arthritis Diet

Anti Inflammatory Recipes to Help with Weight Loss

CONTENTS

INTRODUCTION FROM THE AUTHOR

In 2014 I was finally diagnosed with the debilitating condition of rheumatoid arthritis. The diagnosis took a long time coming, as did any form of medication to counter the condition, and as a result I spent eight months of my life near enough on the sofa at home. I could not walk without crying, my knees and ankles were so badly swollen I could barely get my jeans on and I had no chance of getting any shoes on and I was forced to wear slippers. It is an all too familiar situation for those people unfortunate to suffer from the disease.

During this eight month period when I was existing on concoctions of steroids and pain killers I read every single article I could find on rheumatoid arthritis. Although the final diagnosis took a long time in coming every medical practitioner I saw and every nurse was fairly sure that I did indeed had RA.

During this time it became painfully obvious to me, apologies for the pun, that I was suffering from a western condition brought about by my diet. If you had asked me about my diet before I was diagnosed with RA I would have told you I had a pretty healthy diet. Plenty of fish, loved my smoothies and juices - but I also loved cakes, take away and eating out. So although I did have plenty of healthy food I was also having plenty of unhealthy food, or at least enough to tip the scales in favour or RA.

The more I read the more I had to question what on earth was going on. It seems that the first recorded case of RA in Africa was in the 1960's even though the disease had been around in Europe and recognised since the late 1800's. And that was another thing -

it's a new disease, where did it come from? What was causing it? It is also virtually unknown it appears in countries like South America and Asia, and this made me start to wonder what made me so different from the people in those countries. The answer was of course very simple, diet.

Post my diagnosis I was on a fairly awful set of drugs. Methotrexate was one of these. The drug is I believe is one that they use in chemo-therapy. I would take this, along with a few other drugs on Monday, and I cannot begin to describe how tired it made me feel. I was dogged with a lethargy I just could not shake until about Thursday/Friday when finally I felt a little more alive and motivated, and then all too soon again it was Monday and I would be back at the bottom again. Along with the tiredness were other unpleasant side effects like constant head aches and mouth ulcers. The steroids I had been taken had the unwanted side effect of making me have an over active appetitive, that coupled with the inactivity of sitting on the sofa soon saw the pounds pile on.

My plan became very clear. I wanted to basically feel better, regain control of my life and reduce the medication I was taking. I am not at all advocating you throw away your meds and take into the meal plans that follow as miracle cure for RA. However I've found that I now have a near enough normal life, my joints have been damaged permanently by the disease and there's little I can do about that however the tiredness is a thing of the past, I'm full of energy, back at work, loving the gym and on vastly reduced medication. I put all of this down to the change in my diet and taking time to think about my food choices. Slip ups do occur, I love a take away curry, and from time to time I will have one and boy do I know about it the following day. That in itself however is enough to remind me what life would be like everyday if I ate those kinds of foods again too regularly and it puts me back on the straight and narrow.

The recipes in this book are specifically designed for people with RA who need to eat well and need to loose some weight. Shedding those extra pounds will be a kindness to your aching joints not to mention making you feel better about yourself.

I wish you all the best of luck and hope you can enjoy some of the health benefits I myself have from embracing some new and healthy eating habits.

At the end of this book you will also find a daily planner and exercise record you can use to record your progress.

Ross Lennox

Exercise

We all recognise the important of taking daily exercise and for Rheumatoid Arthritis Sufferers this is especially important. As with all diet and exercise programs it is always advisable to seek medical advice before starting.

When you think about it, the formula for losing weight is pretty simple: calories burned must be greater than consumed ones. In truth, there is an effective way to treat RA and tip the weighing scale to your favor. And, you can do that through exercise.

According to experts, exercise can be seen as a form of medicine without having to take any pills, and for very good reasons. Regular physical activity helps strengthen the bones, lubricates joints, and boosts your energy - and when you are suffering from RA this is just the medicine you need. When you combine a healthy diet with exercise, the pounds disappear even faster than they do with diet alone.

This book will help you make fitness easy and accessible. With the combination of cardio exercises and some strength training, you'll burn calories and melt the fat away.

Incorporating gentle everyday exercise into your daily life can have some wonderful effects. Apart from helping you loose those unwanted pounds and be a trimmer looking you, there are some other super benefits.

Sleep! Do you remember sleep? Do you remember a time when your head hit the pillow and you awoke refreshed and ready for the new day? Rheumatoid Arthritis robbed me peaceful sleep. I would wake myself because of the pain in my joints, the medications seemed to give me hot flushes or I would be feeling so cold I found myself having to hunt out extra covers for the bed. There is no miracle cure for this, but exercise really can help to take the edge off this and promote some restful sleep.

You may not feel like taking any exercise, and I completely understand that when you suffer from RA you lack the energy levels to motivate yourself and the pain you suffer means hitting the gym is the last thing you want to do. However there are things you can do, it is all about taking the very first positive step. A gentle walk perhaps, this not only provides exercise but just getting out the house and changing your environment can be real lift for the spirits. Swimming is really good, and if you can find a swimming pool that has a hot tub why not treat yourself to a soak in there after your swim.

Yoga is the perfect exercise for rheumatoid Arthritis sufferers. You might not feel very flexible now, however a few yoga sessions and you will be surprised how much more supple your body can be.

The Power of Walking

Of all the kinds of physical activity, walking comes most naturally because it's already part of everybody's lives. If you have Rheumatoid Arthritis, a regular walking routine can help slow its progression.

How about weight loss? Indeed, walking can help you reduce pounds and if you have not undertaken any exercise for a long time this is the perfect place to start.

Brisk walking is considered to be an ideal form of aerobic exercise as it is low impact and requires no special equipment other than a good pair of walking shoes. In this exercise program, we'll have 2 kinds of cardio walks.

1. The moderate-intensity pace from beginning to end. This style of walking helps in burning body fat, but is slightly longer than the second type of walk.

2. This is a combination of moderate-intensity pace with intervals, which is short bursts of fast walking. This kind of walk boosts the metabolism for hours even after your workout, so you'll be burning more calories throughout the day.

The table below will help you gauge the speed and intensity of your cardio walks.

Note: Use the speed only as a guide. Remember what feels like a light exercise for one person may be a bit advanced for another.

	Level of Intensity	Speed (MPH)
Warmup and Cooldown	Light (so light that you can still chat with a friend and even sing)	3
Cardio Walks	Moderate (breathing hard but can still talk on your cell phone)	3 ½
Cardio Walks, Intervals	Vigorous (slightly stepping out of your comfort zone)	4-5 +

You may start out with 1 minute at moderate intensity, followed by 30 seconds at vigorous intensity, and then switch between the two. As you progress, you can increase to 1 minute moderate and 1 minute vigorous with 1 minute intervals.

"Be alert to prime drop time" Most exercisers quit within the first few months, especially when they see little results. If you struggle to exercise, find a walking or fitness partner."

This is a sample 10-minute cardio walk that could burn more fats in the process. You may use a stopwatch to time this.

In minutes	Activity	Intensity
0:00	Warmup	4
1:00	Moderate pace	5
4:00	Picking up the pace	6
7:00	Brisk walk, but make sure you're not breathless	7
9:00	Moderate, about to cool down	5-4
10:00	Finish	

On Mastering Cardio Walks

It's imperative that you learn and maintain good form for your cardio walks. Not only to maximize fat burning, but to avoid injury as well - take it easy, listen to your body.

Here's a simple guide to proper walking technique:

- Hold your head high, so the neck and the spine form a straight line. The chin should be level with the ground. Make sure you do not tuck it in towards your neck. The chest should be raised and the shoulders relaxed.

- The arms and hands must be in a proper position, too. Bend the elbows to a 90-degree angle and keep them close to the sides. They should move to the rear, but not outward, as you walk.

- When you step forward, your heel should gently strike the ground before your foot rolls forward and lets you push off from the toes. Do not pound the feet.

- In order to determine the normal length of stride, stand straight and extend one foot a few inches in front of you, with the heels not touching the ground and the legs straight. Then slowly lean forward. That's how far forward your front foot should go during a stride.

- As you walk, your abdominal muscles should be tight. Pull the belly button towards the spine and tuck the pelvis slightly forward. Power your walk from the glutes not on the thighs. You must allow your hips to swing as you walk.
- Finally, as you walk, look ahead of you – at least 10 to 30 feet.

Apart from walking, you may also try these active moves. These are great for lubricating the joints, getting blood flowing to your walking muscles, and reducing the risk of injury. You may do this as an alternative to your walking routine.

1. Hurdles

How to do it: Balance the right leg whilst holding on to a chair for support. Bend the left leg so the heel is behind you. Rotate the leg out to the left side and then forward as if drawing a semi-circle. Do 15 reps on each leg and then switch.

2. Heel raises

Hold on to a chair for support and stand with the feet parallel and hip-width apart. Lift the heels and rise onto your toes for 2 seconds, and then lower. Do 15 reps.

Variation: Do with the heels together and the toes pointing outward.

3. Windmills

Stand with the arms on the sides. Circle the right arm in front of you as though doing the back stroke. Do 15 reps on each arm and then switch.

4. Foot rock overs

Stand with the right foot about 12 inches behind the left foot. The toes on the left should lift off the flow, while the right should be flat on the ground. Shift the weight forward while lowering the left toes and rolling onto the ball of the right foot. Lift the right heel. Go back to starting position. Do 15 reps each and then switch feet.

Do Strength Training

Take the stress off the joints by strengthening the muscles that surround them. It makes sense? With proper form and guidance, strength training could work wonders.

This mini but effective strength training is for people with Rheumatoid Arthritis and delivers a multitude of benefits. Some of them are:

- Strength training builds the muscles, which burns more calories than fat does. This means that the more muscles you have, the more calories you burn even while you sleep.

- Strength training tones and firms both the upper and lower body. You can modify the exercises below and choose just 4 to make it less challenging if you are just starting out with exercise. Just remember to do the version of each move depending on your fitness level.

- Strength training is a kind of weight-bearing activity that builds bone density and protects against bone-thinning diseases such as osteoporosis, arthritis, and the like.

These exercises can be performed 2 or 3 days a week.

✓ Pendulum kickback – this tones the triceps and thighs

How to do it: Hold a dumbbell in each hand. Stand with the left leg straight in front of you. Bend the elbows to a 90-degree angle so that the forearms are parallel to the floor. Swing the left leg behind and squeeze the glutes as you straighten the arms. Return to starting position. Do 12 reps and then switch legs.

✓ 4-SquatCurl – this tones the biceps and thighs

How to do it: Hold a dumbbell in your left hand at your side. Cross the right ankle over the left thigh. Bend the left knee and hip. Sit back, keeping the knee behind the toes. As you do this, raise the dumbbell to the left shoulder. Return to starting position. Do 12 reps before switching sides.

✓ Leg kick

How to do it: lie on the right side with the legs straight and together, similar to a long line position. Prop up the right elbow and forearm, lifting the ribs off the floor and the head towards the ceiling. Place the left hand lightly on the floor in front of you. Raise the left leg to hip level and flex the foot pointing forward. Exhale as you swing the left leg forward. 1 rep should be: inhale, point toes, and swing leg backward past the right leg.

✓ Crouch and Pull – this tones the shoulders, arms, oblique, and upper back

How to do it: Hold a dumbbell in each hand, stand with the feet shoulder-width apart, and sit back to a partial squat. Hinge forward from the hips whilst keeping the arms extended below the shoulders and the palms facing in. With the lower body facing forward, rotate the torso to the left. Bend the left arm and pull the dumbbell towards the chest, pointing the elbow towards the ceiling. Return to starting position and then repeat alternating sides.

✓ Liftoff Lunge – this tones the shoulders, triceps, and thighs

How to do it: stand with feet-width apart. Hold dumbbells at shoulders with the palms facing forward. Step back with the right foot, bend both knees, and then lower yourself until the left thigh is parallel to the floor. Press into the left foot and stand up as you pull the right knee forward, keeping the balance on the left leg. Raise the weights overhead and switch the right leg back into lunge position as you lower the weights. Return to starting position and then repeat alternating sides.

✓ Knee-hugger Chest Fly – this tones the chest and abdominals

How to do it: hold a dumbbell in each hand, lie faceup with the knees bent and the shins parallel to the floor. The arms should be put to the sides with the elbows slightly bent and the palms facing up. Contract the abdominal muscles and lift the hips off the floor, about 3 inches. While doing so, squeeze the chest muscles and raise your arms, bringing the dumbbells together over the chest. Lower arms and hips to the starting position and then repeat.

Sample Workout for Weeks 1 to 4

	Week 1	Week 2	Week 3	Week 4
Day 1	Moderate-intensity walk, 20	Moderate-intensity walk, 25 mins.	Moderate-intensity walk, 30 mins.	Moderate-intensity walk, 35 mins.

	mins.			
Day 2	Strength training, choose any 4 exercises above	Strength training, choose any 4-5 exercises above	Strength training, choose any 5-6 exercises above	Strength training, perform all 6 exercises above
Day 3	Moderate-intensity with intervals, 15 mins	Moderate-intensity with intervals, 20 mins	Strength training, choose any 4-5 exercises above	Strength training, choose any 5 exercises above
Day 4	Rest	Moderate-intensity walk, 25 mins.	Moderate-intensity walk, 30 mins.	Rest
Day 5	Moderate-intensity walk, 20 mins.	Rest	Rest	Moderate-intensity walk, 35 mins.
Day 6	Strength training, choose any 4 exercises above	Strength training, choose any 5 exercises above	Moderate-intensity with intervals, 25 mins	Moderate-intensity with intervals, 30 mins
Day 7	Moderate-intensity with intervals, 15 mins	Moderate-intensity with intervals, 20 mins	Strength training, choose any 5 exercises above	Strength training, perform all 6 exercises above

"Treat yourself every once in a while. To celebrate your commitment to fitness, treat yourself to a little something at the end of each workout week. This can be as simple as a massage, a new outfit, or anything that can make you feel all the more motivated."

Best Vegetables for Rheumatoid Arthritis

Going green – and orange and yellow vegetables – when you have rheumatoid arthritis could do your joints a big favor. When you're suffering from arthritis, filling your pantry with fresh produce is one of the most important things to do. This is because vegetables are rich in important nutrients and antioxidants that lower inflammation and shield against cell damage. According to nutritionists, colorful vegetables are the best.

The following vegetables should color your dishes every day.

Red and Green Peppers
No matter the color, peppers are known to be rich in vitamin C, which helps protect bones and the cells in the cartilage.

Dark Green Leafy Vegetables
Green, leafy vegetables such as Brussel sprouts, kale, broccoli, bok choy, spinach, and Swiss chard are loaded with antioxidants that protect the cells from free-radicals. These are also high in calcium.

Garlic, Onions, Shallots, and Leeks
These vegetables are packed with quercetin, a type of antioxidant that has the ability to relieve inflammation and reduces enzymes damaging the cartilage.

Sweet Potatoes, Carrots, Red Peppers and Squash
These vegetables are also rich in antioxidants and in beta-cryptoxanthin that could lessen the risk of developing arthritis and other related inflammatory ailments.

Best Fruits for Rheumatoid Arthritis

Fruits offer an extensive dosage of fiber, vitamins, minerals, and antioxidants that lower inflammation and help get rid of free radicals.

Olives
Olives can be powerful inflammation fighters. Similar to that of extra-virgin olive oil that contains a natural anti-inflammatory agent.

Strawberries
Strawberries have more vitamin C than oranges and are low in sugar. Vitamin C can lower the possibility of gout and arthritis flares.

Avocado
The fruit has high content of anti-inflammatory monounsaturated fat and is rich in carotenoid lutein. A diet rich in avocado decreases the risk of joint damage in early osteoarthritis.

Grapes
These are a great source of polyphenols and antioxidants. They are also a potent anti-inflammatory that help in improving the symptoms of osteoarthritis.

Fish

Best Fish for Rheumatoid Arthritis

According to research, those who eat fish on a regular basis are less likely to develop arthritis because it contains omega-3s. Some of the allowed fish for this diet include: Salmon, mackerel, sardines, tuna, herring, black cod, and lake trout.

Best Seeds and Nuts for Rheumatoid Arthritis

Nuts are rich in vitamin E, magnesium, and larginine that help keep body inflammation under control. Some examples include - peanuts, walnuts, pistachios, almonds, chia seeds, and flax seeds.

Best Grains for Rheumatoid Arthritis

In order to minimize inflammation and maximize health and nutrition, you should stock on whole gluten-free grains. These are rich in antioxidants and B vitamins that protect cell damage. Some examples include barley, bulgur, amaranth, quinoa, brown rice, millet, whole oats, and rye.

Best Spices for Rheumatoid Arthritis

Following an arthritis diet would mean choosing the right condiments and spices as well. Some of the spices include:

Garlic
Garlic contains an anti-inflammatory compound called diallyl disulfide that controls pro-inflammatory cytokines effects. This also helps fight inflammation and pain caused by arthritis.

Ginger
There are chemicals found in ginger known as shogaol and Gingerol that block inflammation pathways. This herb is also rich in anti-inflammatory properties and lessens the symptoms of osteoarthritis symptoms.

Turmeric
The active chemical called curcumin is contained in the turmeric root that prevents inflammatory enzymes and cytokines in two inflammatory pathways. This helps reduce swelling and joint pain as well.

Cayenne
Cayenne contain scapsaicinoids, a natural compound that has anti-inflammatory properties.

Cinnamon
Cinnamon has antioxidant properties called cinnamic acid and cinnamaldehyde that help hinder cell damage. Use this in combination with other spices and it may provide cumulative anti-inflammatory effects.

Food to Avoid

Processed Food

Ready to eat and those that are from a packet should not be part of your rheumatoid arthritis diet. This is because these food are packed with preservatives, sugar, salt, and additives to increase shelf-life. Too much of these are bad for everyone's health and could lead to inflammation and flare ups.

Sugar and Refined Carbs

Foods that are filled with these cause a sugar spike that produce cytokines, a pro-inflammatory chemical that worsens arthritis joint pain.

Red Meat

This causes the body's inflammatory response thereby increasing pain and swelling in joints. In fact, those who are suffering from rheumatoid arthritis noticed great improvement in their symptoms when they give up meat and modify their diet to plant-based proteins such as soy, legumes, and beans.

Fried Food

Food cooked this way leads to us ingesting harmful compounds known as AGEs or Glycation End products (AGEs) that are connected to inflammation and oxidative stress. If you're going to fry your food, make sure to use healthy oils.

Gluten

According to research, rheumatoid arthritis has a genetic connection with other autoimmune diseases. That is why you needs to cut back on glutens that are hard to digest and could contribute to inflammation.

Dairy

A protein found in milk called casein could cause flare ups, and vitamin D found in dairy products is negatively linked with arthritis.

Breakfast Recipes

Spinach and Tofutti Cheese Frittata

Ingredients:

For the frittata
- 1 tbsp. olive oil
- 1 onion, sliced
- 1 garlic clove, minced
- 1 cup spinach
- 1 cup applesauce
- 1/3 cup coconut milk
- ½ cup Tofutti cheese

For the Salsa
- 1 garlic clove, minced
- 2 green onions, minced
- 4 tomatoes, chopped
- 2 tbsp. fresh cilantro, minced
- ¼ tsp. salt
- 1/8 tsp. pepper

Directions:
1. Preheat the oven to 350 F. pour olive oil in a skillet.
2. Once the oil is hot, sauté onion and garlic for 3 minutes or until translucent and aromatic. Add in spinach.
3. Meanwhile, combine applesauce and coconut milk in a bowl. Whisk until frothy.
4. Pour mixture over spinach. Cook for 7 minutes. Sprinkle cheese.
5. Place inside the oven and bake for 10 minutes.
6. For the salsa, put together garlic, onions, cilantro, tomatoes, salt, and pepper in a bowl. Pour over frittata. Serve.

Toasted Egg Rolls

Ingredients:

- Wholemeal bread, sliced thinly, crust removed
- ½ oz olive oil
- 2 eggs
- Pinch of salt
- Pinch of pepper
- 1 tbsp. skimmed milk

Directions:

1. Melt olive oil in a pan. Pour eggs and then the milk. Season with salt and pepper. Whisk well.
2. Pour scrambled egg over the bread.
3. Roll up and cook for 2 minutes. Serve.

Oat Milk Jelly with Berries

Oat milk jelly
- coconut oil, for greasing
- 2 pouches unflavored gelatin, preferably 7 grams each
- 2 tsp. palm sugar, crumbled
- 2 cups oat milk, unsweetened
- 2 cups water
- ½ tsp. vanilla extract

Fruit salad
- 1 cup strawberries
- 1 cup raspberries
- 1 cup blackberries

Directions:
1. Lightly grease a baking dish with coconut oil.
2. Put together gelatin, sugar, oat milk, and water in a saucepan. Stir mixture or until the gelatin dissolves.
3. Allow to simmer whilst stirring continuously. You will know that the gelatin is done the moment it sticks to the back of the spoon. Turn off the heat. Stir in vanilla extract.
4. Pour gelatin into the baking dish. Allow to cool slightly at room temperature before sealing with saran wrap. Place inside the fridge to chill for 2-4 hours before slicing into bite-sized cubes.
5. For the salad, put together strawberries, raspberries, and black berries into a bowl. Tip in cubed gelatin. Toss to combine.
6. To serve, ladle equal amounts into bowls. Serve.

Breakfast Spiced Omelette

Ingredients:

For the Sauce
- 1 Tbsp. cornstarch
- 2 Tbsp. water
- 1 cup chicken stock, low-sodium
- 2 tsp. rice wine vinegar
- 1 Tbsp. light soy sauce
- 2 tsp. palm sugar, crumbled
- Pinch of sea salt
- Pinch of white pepper

Omelette
- 6 eggs, lightly whisked
- ½ cup sweet ham, cooked, diced
- 1 cup bean sprouts
- ¼ tsp. red pepper flakes
- ¼ cup cabbage
- 4 water chestnuts, minced
- 1 tsp. light soy sauce
- 2 tsp. coconut oil, divided
- ¼ cup scallions, minced, for garnish

Directions:
1. Dissolve cornstarch in water. Stir. Set aside.
2. Meanwhile, combine chicken stock, rice wine vinegar, soy sauce, palm sugar, salt, and white pepper in to the saucepan. Pour in corn starch.
3. Stir and cook until the sauce thickens. Turn off the heat.
4. For the omelet, combine eggs, sweet ham, bean sprouts, red pepper flakes, napa cabbage, water chestnuts, light soy sauce in a large bowl. Mix.
5. Heat the coconut oil in a non-stick skillet. Pour just the right amount of the mixture. Cook egg until partially set. Flip. Cook the other side for 1 minute.
6. Transfer to a plate. Cook remaining egg mixture. Garnish with fresh scallions. Serve with the sauce on the side.

Apple, Avocado, and Carrot Salad with Curry Vinaigrette

Vinaigrette
- 1 garlic clove, quartered
- 1 shallot, minced
- 2 Tbsp. curry powder
- Pinch of sea salt
- Pinch of black pepper to taste
- 1 Tbsp. garam masala
- 3 Tbsp. apple cider vinegar
- 3 Tbsp. pomegranate vinegar
- ¼ cup extra virgin olive oil

Salad
- 2 apples, sliced thinly
- ¼ lb. baby spinach leaves, rinsed, spun-dried
- 1 lb. baby carrots, boiled in salted water until tender
- 1 avocados, sliced into chunks

Directions:
1. Combine garlic clove, shallot, curry powder, salt, black pepper, garam masala, apple cider vinegar, pomegranate vinegar, and extra virgin olive oil. Whisk all ingredients come together and the salt dissolves.
2. Place apples, baby spinach leaves, baby carrots, and avocados in a salad bowl. Drizzle in half of the dressing. Gently toss to combine.
3. To serve, spoon salad into plates. Season with just the right amount of vinaigrette.

Baguette Stuffed with Chicken Salad

Ingredients:
- 1 gluten-free baguette
- 4 servings Chicken Salad, this can be store-bought or homemade
- 1 ½ Tbsp. English mustard, for spreading

Directions:
1. To make the sandwich, spread mustard on one part of the bread.
2. Stuff with chicken salad. Slice bread into equal portions. Serve.

Broccoli on Apple Cider Vinegar and Maple Syrup

Ingredients:

- 5 cups broccoli florets
- 1/3 cup water
- 1 tsp. olive oil
- 1 tbsp. maple syrup
- 1 tbsp. apple cider vinegar
- Pinch of salt
- Pinch of pepper
- ¼ cup pumpkin seeds

Directions:

1. Pour water in a skillet. Bring to a boil. Add in broccoli florets. Cook for 3 minutes, covered.
2. Cook, uncovered, for another 3 minutes or until the broccoli is tender and the water evaporates.
3. Meanwhile, pour olive oil into the skillet. Stir in broccoli for 2 minutes. Remove from heat. Transfer to a serving dish.
4. Drizzle broccoli with maple syrup and apple cider vinegar. Season with salt and red pepper. Scatter pumpkin seeds on top.

Gluten-free Rolls Stuffed with Vegetable Salad

Ingredients:
- 4 servings vegetable salad, either store-bought or homemade
- 1 Tbsp. English mustard, for spreading

For the bread

Dry ingredients
- 1 cup almond flour, finely milled
- 1 ½ Tbsp. instant bread yeast
- 2 tsp. xanthan gum
- ½ cup tapioca flour
- 1 ½ cup sweet potato starch
- 1 Tbsp. palm sugar, crumbled
- 1 ½ tsp. sea salt

Wet ingredients
- 1 cup warm water
- 3 egg whites, whisked
- 1 tsp. coconut vinegar
- 1 Tbsp. coconut oil

Directions:
1. Preheat the oven to 425°F. Lightly grease baking sheet with parchment paper; e with coconut oil.
2. To make the bread, put together almond flour, instant bread yeast, xanthan gum, tapioca flour, sweet potato starch, palm sugar, and sea salt in a mixing bowl.
3. Create a well in the center. Pour warm water, egg whites, coconut vinegar, and coconut oil
4. Mix until the dough comes together. Set aside dough for 15 minutes.
5. Divide into equal portions. Place dough in a floured surface and shape into balls.
6. Set aside dough for another 15 minutes.
7. Place on a baking sheet and bake for 30 minutes or until the crust is golden brown and the loaf risen.

8.   Remove baking sheet from the oven. Let cool ion a cake rack. Slice off ½ inch off the bread and scoop out just the right amount of bread filling.

9.   To make the sandwich, spread mustard on scooped out part of the bread. Stuff salad into bread. Serve.

Stuffed Eggs with Mushrooms

Ingredients:

- ½ cup mushrooms, chopped
- Olive oil
- 2 tsp. parsley
- 3 eggs, hard-boiled, halved
- Worcester sauce
- 1 cup cottage cheese

Directions:

1. Baste mushrooms with olive oil. Sauté together with parsley.
2. Remove yolk from the egg and mash. Combine Worcester sauce.
3. Fill the egg whites with stuffing. Put cottage cheese on top. Grill for 3 minutes.

Avocado Spinach Spread

Ingredients:
- Gluten-free bread, toasted
- Olive oil
- 2 cups spinach
- Pinch of sea salt
- Pinch of ground black pepper
- ½ avocado, flesh scooped out, mashed
- 1 tomato, sliced into rounds
- 2 eggs, poached

Directions:
1. Pour olive oil in a nonstick skillet. Once the oil is hot, cook spinach for 2 minutes or until wilted.
2. Place spinach into a mesh. Allow to cool before squeezing out excess liquid.
3. Transfer to a plate. Season with salt and pepper.
4. Spread mashed avocado on toasted bread. Put tomato slices on top and spinach. Add in eggs. Serve.

Oatmeal Pancakes

Ingredients:

- 8 tbsp. rolled oats
- 1 oz plain flour
- 1 egg, beaten
- 1 tsp. honey
- Olive oil
- ½ pint skimmed milk

Directions:

1. Put together oats and flour in a bowl. Add in egg and drizzle in honey.
2. Pour the egg-honey mixture into the oats-flour mix. Stir in milk.
3. Meanwhile, heat the oil in a pan. Pour just the right amount of the batter mixture. Cook until the side is golden brown and the top set.
4. Flip and cook the other side for another minute.
5. Transfer to a serving dish. Drizzle in honey. Serve.

Chive Flat Bread

Ingredients:

- ½ cup coconut oil, melted
- 4 cups almond flour, finely milled
- ½ cup fresh chives, minced
- 2 ½ cups water
- Pinch of kosher salt

Dipping sauce

- sweet chili sauce

Directions:

1. Lightly grease a non-stick skillet with coconut oil. Set aside.
2. Put together almond flour, chives, water, and salt in a bowl. Mix until the dough comes together.
3. On a lightly floured flat surface, turn out the dough and knead until elastic.
4. Roll into balls, tucking in edges underneath. Flatten using a rolling pin.
5. In a skillet, fry flat breads until small pockets of air develops within. Flip to the other side. Cook until light brown on both sides.
6. Transfer to a serving platter. Lightly grease both sides of the flat bread with oil. Cover platter with tea towel sot eh bread won't dry out. Repeat the same cooking procedure until all flat breads are cooked.
7. Serve with desired amount of sweet chili sauce on the side.

Greens and Reds Salad

Ingredients:

For the Dressing
- 1 tsp. extra virgin olive oil
- 3 tsp. apple cider vinegar
- 1 tsp. palm sugar, crumbled
- Pinch of salt
- Pinch of white pepper

- 2 red apples, diced
- 10 green grapes, quartered
- ¼ cup roasted walnuts, lightly salted

Directions:
1. Put together palm sugar, salt, white pepper, apple cider vinegar, and extra virgin olive oil in a bottle with tight fitting lid. Seal and shake well until ingredients dissolve.
2. Mix red apples, green grapes, and walnuts in a salad bowl. Drizzle in just the right amount of dressing. Toss well.
3. Place equal portions into salad bowls. Serve.

Artichoke Hearts Soup

Ingredients:

- 1 can artichoke hearts, quartered
- 2 cups vegetable broth, divided
- ¼ tsp. xanthan gum
- 2 tbsp. non-dairy butter
- 1 garlic clove, minced
- ½ onion, minced
- 1 celery stalk, diced
- 2 handfuls spinach leaves
- 1 tbsp. lemon juice, freshly squeezed
- Pinch of salt
- Pinch of ground black pepper
- ½ cup non-dairy cream

Directions:

1. Place artichoke hearts in a food processor. Pour ¼ cup of vegetable broth together with xanthan gum. Process until pureed.

2. Meanwhile, place butter in a non-stick skillet. Sauté garlic, onion, and celery until onion becomes tender and the garlic fragrant.

3. Spoon artichoke puree, add then pour the remaining broth and spinach leaves. Let it simmer for 10 minutes or until the spinach wilts.

4. Add in lemon juice and cream. Season with salt and pepper. You can either serve immediately or chilled.

Apple and Butternut Squash Soup

Ingredients:

- 1 lb butternut squash
- 1 tbsp. olive oil
- 1 cup non-dairy milk
- 1 onion, chopped
- 1 ½ tsp. ginger, grated
- 2 apples, diced
- ½ tsp. cumin
- ¾ tsp. curry powder
- Pinch of salt
- Pinch of black pepper
- 3 cups vegetable broth

Directions:
1. Preheat the oven to 375 degrees F.
2. Prepare a sheet of aluminium foil big enough to wrap the squash. Place inside the oven and bake for 30 minutes.
3. Remove from the oven. Set aside to cool. Once cooled, peel squash and remove the seeds.
4. Dice squash. Transfer to a food processor. Pour milk and process until smooth. Transfer to a bowl. Set aside.
5. Meanwhile, heat the olive oil in a saucepan. Once hot, sauté onion, ginger, apples, curry powder, cumin, and vegetable broth. Season with salt and black pepper.
6. Bring mixture to a boil. Once boiling, let it simmer for 8 minutes. Turn off the heat.
7. Set aside to cool before transferring to a food processor. Puree until smooth.
8. Pour pureed mixture back into the saucepan. Add in butternut squash mixture. Allow to simmer over medium flame.
9. Adjusting taste, if needed. Serve immediately.

Grilled Mushrooms

Ingredients:

- Olive oil
- 1 cup mushrooms of choice, washed, stalks and skin removed
- Pinch of sea salt
- Pinch of pepper
- Nutmeg
- 2 whole meal toast

Directions:

1. Baste mushrooms with olive oil. Season with nutmeg, salt, and pepper.
2. Place mushrooms in the barbecue grill. Grill for 8 minutes.
3. Serve with whole meal toast.

Coconut Porridge with Cocoa

Ingredients:
- ¼ cup rolled oats
- ½ cup coconut milk
- 1 tbsp. cocoa powder
- 1¼ cups water
- 1 tsp. palm sugar, crumbled
- 1 tbsp. cashew nuts, toasted

Directions:
1. Place rolled oats, coconut milk, cocoa powder, water, and palm sugar into the Dutch oven. Stir mixture well.
2. Bring to a boil. Turn down heat.
3. Once boiling, allow to simmer for 20 minutes, stirring occasionally. Turn off the heat immediately. Adjust taste if needed.
4. To serve, ladle equal amounts of porridge into bowls. Cool slightly before serving.

Banana Pancakes

Ingredients:

- 2 tsp. baking powder
- 1 cup flour
- 1 ½ cups soy milk, divided
- 1 banana, mashed
- 1 tbsp. sweetener
- Sliced fruits of choice, for garnish
- Olive oil

Directions:

1. Sift together baking powder and flour in a bowl.

2. In a separate bowl, pour ¼ cup of soy milk and banana. Mix well. Add in sweetener and the remaining milk. Stir.

3. In a non-stick skillet, heat the oil. Once hot, pour 1 cup of batter. Cook until the edges are golden brown and the center is no longer runny. Flip the pancake over and cook the other side for another minute.

4. Repeat the process until all batter is cooked. Garnish with fresh fruit of choice. Serve.

Lunch Recipes

Vegetable Casserole

Ingredients:
- 1 tbsp.olive oil
- 1 garlic clove, crushed
- 2 leeks, sliced
- 3 celery sticks, chopped
- 1 lb tomatoes, chopped
- 2 carrots, sliced
- 1 sweet potato, diced
- ¾ cup brown lentils
- 2 parsnips, diced
- 1 rutabaga, diced
- 1 tbsp. thyme, chopped
- 1 tbsp. fresh marjoram, chopped
- 3 cups vegetable stock
- 3 tbsp. water
- 1 tbsp. corn flour
- Pinch of salt
- Pinch of ground black pepper
- Fresh thyme sprigs, for garnish

Directions
1. Preheat the oven to 350 degrees F.
2. Pour olive oil in an oven-safe casserole. Sauté garlic, leeks, and celery for 3 minutes or until tender.
3. Add in tomatoes, carrots, sweet potatoes, lentils, parsnips, rutabaga, thyme, and marjoram. Pour vegetable stock. Stir. Bring mixture to a boil.
4. Place casserole inside the oven. Bake for 50 minutes. Remove casserole from the oven.
5. Put together water and corn flour in a bowl. Pour over the casserole. Season with salt and pepper.
6. Place casserole on a stovetop and heat for 3 minutes or until the sauce thickens over low flame.
7. To serve, ladle into bowls. Garnish with thyme sprigs.

Spinach and Grape Tomatoes Salad

Ingredients:
- 4 tsp. balsamic vinegar
- 2 tsp. vegetable oil
- 1 ½ tsp. sugar
- Dash of Worcestershire sauce
- 2 cups spinach
- ½ cup grape tomatoes
- 1 oz. Tofutti cheese

Directions:
1. Put together balsamic vinegar, vegetable oil, sugar, and Worcestershire sauce in a bowl. Mix well. Set aside.
2. Put spinach and grape tomatoes in a bowl.
3. Pour dressing all over the vegetables. Put tofutti cheese on top. Serve.

Yang Chow Veggie Rice

Ingredients:

- 2 tbsp.olive oil
- 1 onion, diced
- 4 garlic cloves, chopped
- ¼ cup tomatoes, diced
- 4 cups brown rice, leftover will do
- ½ cup green peas
- ½ cup carrots, diced
- 1 cup tofu, mashed
- ½ cup cabbage, shredded
- 1 tbsp. soy sauce
- Pinch of salt
- Pinch of pepper

Directions:

1. Pour olive oil in a non-stick skillet. Sauté onion, garlic, and tomatoes for 4 minutes. Tip in leftover brown rice and green peas.

2. Stir continuously until all ingredients come together. Add in carrots, tofu, and cabbage into the mix.

3. Meanwhile, combine soy sauce, salt, and pepper in a small bowl. Pour over the rice mixture. Continue stirring until everything is cooked through. Serve.

Spinach Tofu Scramble

Ingredients:

- ½ tbsp. olive oil
- 1 onion, minced
- ½ tsp. garlic, minced
- ½ bell pepper, minced
- 8 oz extra firm tofu, crumbled
- ½ cup spinach
- ½ tsp. paprika
- ½ tsp. cumin
- ¼ tsp. turmeric
- 1 tbsp. nutritional yeast
- Pinch of sea salt
- Pinch of ground black pepper

Directions:

1. Pour olive oil in a non-stick skillet. Sauté onion, garlic, and bell pepper for 3 minutes or until aromatic and tender.
2. Add in crumbled tofu in the skillet. Sauté until all ingredients are mixed. Tip in spinach.
3. Season with paprika, cumin, turmeric, salt, and pepper. Stir in nutritional yeast. Continue mixing until cooked through. Serve.

Broccoli Matchsticks

Ingredients:
- 2 broccoli stems, sliced into thick matchsticks
- olive oil, for shallow frying
- 1 cup almond milk
- 1 cup almond flour, finely milled
- Pinch of salt
- Dash of Spanish paprika
- ¼ cup cashew cheese

Directions:
1. Pour olive oil into a non-stick skillet.
2. Place almond milk, almond flour, and breading in 3 different bowls.
3. Dredge broccoli matchstick in this order: flour, milk. Repeat until all matchsticks are breaded.
4. Once the oil is hot, fry broccoli matchsticks until crisp and golden brown. Drain on paper towels.
5. Season with salt and paprika. Serve with cashew cheese as dip.

Cauliflower Casserole

Ingredients:
- Olive oil
- 1 garlic clove, chopped
- 1 onion, chopped
- ½ cup green bell pepper, chopped
- ¼ cup celery, sliced thinly
- 3 cups cauliflower, chopped
- 1 tbsp. balsamic vinegar
- 1/8 tsp. salt
- 1/8 tsp. ground black pepper

Directions:
1. Heat the olive oil in a non-stick pan. Sauté onion, garlic, celery, and bell pepper for 5 minutes or until tender.
2. Add in cauliflower. Pour balsamic vinegar. Season with salt and pepper.
3. Bring mixture to a boil. Once boiling, reduce to a simmer for 10 minutes. Serve.

Sweet Corn and Chipotle Chowder

Ingredients:

- 1 tbsp. coconut oil
- 2 garlic cloves, minced
- 1 cup onion, diced
- ½ cup carrot, diced
- ½ cup celery, diced
- 1 sweet potato, diced
- Pinch of sea salt
- Pinch of ground black pepper
- 2 cups sweet corn kernels, fresh
- 1 ½ tbsp. chipotle pepper in sauce, minced
- 1 cup coconut milk
- 3 cups vegetable broth
- ¼ cup red bell pepper
- ½ tbsp. parsley, chopped
- ¼ tsp. cilantro, chopped

Directions:

1. Pour coconut oil in a non-stick pan. Sauté garlic, onion, carrot, and celery until tender and fragrant.
2. Add in sweet potato. Season with salt and pepper. Sauté until the potatoes are tender.
3. Stir in corn kernels and chipotle peppers. Stir well. Pour coconut milk and vegetable broth. Bring mixture to boil.
4. Once boiling, reduce the heat and allow to simmer for 10 minutes.
5. Let cool before transferring to an immersion blender. Blend to the desired level of consistency.
6. Transfer back to the pan. Tip in red bell pepper, parsley, and cilantro. Heat for 2 minutes. Serve.

Cauliflower and Carrots Rice

Ingredients:
- 2 cups brown rice
- 1 garlic clove, minced
- 1 tsp. ginger, grated
- 1 shallot, minced
- 1 carrot, diced
- 1 cauliflower, sliced into bite-sized florets
- 1 tbsp. curry powder
- 1 can coconut cream
- Pinch of salt
- 4 cups vegetable stock

Directions:
1. Pour brown rice, garlic clove, ginger, shallot, carrot, cauliflower, curry powder, coconut cream, and salt in the rice cooker.
2. Pour vegetable stock. Stir. Close the lid. Press the "cook" button of the rice cooker and just wait for the machine to automatically shift to warm.
3. To serve, ladle just the right portions in bowls. Serve.

Halibut Fillets on Bed of Fresh Greens

Ingredients:
- 4 halibut fillets, trimmed well
- Pinch of salt
- Pinch of pepper
- 2 tbsp. sesame oil

For the Dressing
- 2 tsp. sesame oil
- 1 tsp. garlic, grated
- 1 tsp. yellow mustard
- 1 tsp. ginger, grated
- ½ tsp. honey
- ¼ cup lime juice, freshly squeezed

For the Salad
- ¼ lb asparagus, drained
- 1 cabbage, julienned
- 1 cucumber, thinly sliced
- ¼ lb snap beans, drained
- 1 red chilli, minced
- ¼ cup mint leaves
- ¼ cup coriander leaves

Directions:
1. Season halibut fillets with salt, pepper, and sesame. Grill for 4 minutes on each sides. Transfer grilled fillets to aluminium foil sheets. Let sit for 5 minutes.
2. To make the dressing, put together mustard, ginger, garlic, yellow honey, lime juice, and sesame oil in a tight-fitting bottle. Shake well.
3. To make the salad, combine asparagus, cabbage, cucumber, snap beans, red chilli, mint leaves, and coriander leaves in a salad bowl. Drizzle half the dressing all over. Toss well to combine.
4. To serve, portion salad in plates. Place halibut fillets on top. Drizzle unjust the right amount of dressing.

Braised Courgettes and Aubergines

Ingredients:
- 1 aubergine, cut into ½ inch slices
- 2 courgettes, sliced into triangular wedge
- 1 tbsp. olive oil
- 2 garlic cloves, chopped finely
- 1 onion, diced
- 2 red chillies, chopped finely
- 1 tbsp. black bean sauce
- 3 tbsp. water
- Pinch of salt
- Pinch of pepper

Directions:
1. Layer aubergine in a colander. Season with salt. Leave aubergine in the colander for 25 minutes to drain.
2. After 25 minutes, rinse aubergine under cold running water. Drain thoroughly on kitchen paper.
3. Meanwhile, heat the olive oil in a pan. Sauté garlic, onion, and chillies. Sauté for 3 minutes. Tip in black bean sauce. Toss well.
4. Reduce the heat. Add the aubergine into the mixture and sauté for 2 minutes.
5. Add in courgettes and water. Season with salt and pepper. Serve.

Spicy Coconut Mushrooms

Ingredients:
- 2 tbsp.olive oil
- 2 onions, chopped finely
- 2 garlic cloves, chopped finely
- 2 red chillies, sliced into rings
- 2 cups brown cap mushrooms, thickly sliced
- 2/3 cup coconut milk
- Pinch of salt
- Pinch of ground black pepper
- 2 tbsp. coriander, chopped

Directions
1. Pour olive oil in a nonstick pan. Sauté onion, garlic, and, chillies for 4 minutes or until tender and aromatic. Add in brown cap mushrooms. cook for 4 minutes.
2. Pour coconut milk. Bring mixture to a boil. Season with salt and pepper.
3. Garnish with coriander before serving.

Kidney Beans Curry

Ingredients:
- 2 tbsp. olive oil
- ½ tsp. cumin seeds
- 1 onion, sliced thinly
- 2 garlic cloves, crushed
- 1 inch root ginger, grated
- 1 green chilli, chopped finely
- ½ tsp. chili powder
- 1 tsp. ground coriander
- 2 tbsp. curry paste
- Pinch of salt
- Pinch of pepper
- 1 can red kidney beans
- 1 can tomatoes, chopped
- 2 tbsp. fresh coriander, chopped

Directions:
1. Heat the olive oil in a pan. Once hot, sauté cumin seeds for 2 minutes. Add in onion, garlic, ginger, and green chili for 4 minutes.
2. Tip in chilli powder, coriander, curry paste, salt, and pepper. Cook for 5 minutes.
3. Add in kidney beans, tomatoes, and coriander to the pan. Cover and cook for 20 minutes.
4. Adjust seasoning, if needed. Garnish with fresh coriander. Serve.

Pepper and Tomatoes Casserole

Ingredients:
- Olive oil
- 1 onion, chopped
- 1 garlic clove, chopped
- ¼ cup celery, thinly sliced
- ½ cup green bell pepper, chopped
- 3 cups tomatoes, chopped
- 1 tbsp. balsamic vinegar
- 1/8 tsp. salt
- 1/8 tsp. ground black pepper

Directions:
1. Pour olive oil in a nonstick pan. Sauté onion, garlic, celery, and green bell pepper for 5 minutes or until tender and fragrant.
2. Add in tomatoes. Pour balsamic vinegar. Season with salt and pepper.
3. Bring mixture to a boil. Once boiling, allow to simmer for 10 minutes. Serve.

Lemon Brown Rice

Ingredients:
- 1 tbsp. extra-virgin olive oil
- 4 cups leeks
- 1 cup carrots, diced
- 1 tsp. dried oregano
- 1 cup brown rice
- 1 tbsp. chicken stock
- 2 cups water
- 2 tbsp. lemon juice, freshly squeezed
- 2 tbsp. lemon zest, grated
- Pinch of salt
- Pinch of white pepper

Directions:
1. Pour olive oil in a saucepan, heat the olive oil. Sauté leeks, carrots, and dried oregano for 5 minutes or until tender.
2. Add in brown rice. Cook for 1 minute. Stir continuously.
3. Pour chicken stock and water. Bring mixture to a boil. Once boiling, reduce to a simmer for 15 minutes.
4. Remove from the saucepan. Let dish sit for another 2 minutes.
5. Pour lemon juice and zest. Season with salt and white pepper. Serve.

Grilled Chicken Cajun on Bed of Greens

Ingredients:
- 1 tsp. onion powder
- 4 tbsp. salad oil
- Pinch of salt
- Pinch of pepper
- 4 chicken breast halves
- 4 cups mixed salad greens
- 1 carrot, chopped
- 1 red sweet pepper
- 1 green onion, chopped

For the Dressing
- ½ cup salad oil
- 1 tbsp. apple cider vinegar
- 1 tbsp. mustard
- 1 tbsp. water
- 1 tsp. onion powder
- 1 tsp. garlic powder
- 1 tsp. thyme

Directions:
1. Preheat the grill to 170 degrees F.
2. Meanwhile, combine onion powder, salad oil, salt, and pepper in a bowl. Mix well.
3. Baste chicken with the mixture. Grill for 15 minutes on both sides.
4. In a salad bowl, put together salad greens, carrot, red sweet pepper, and onion.
5. To make the dressing, combine salad oil, apple cider vinegar, mustard, water, onion powder, garlic powder, and thyme in a jar with tight-fitting lid. Shake well.
6. To serve, portion salad in plates. Place grilled chicken on top. Drizzle in just the right amount of dressing.

Cold Asparagus Salad

Ingredients:
- 2 ½ lbs. white asparagus, halved, bottoms and tops separated
- water, for boiling

For the Sauce
- 1 tsp. palm sugar, crumbled
- 2 tbsp. light soy sauce
- Pinch of Himalayan pink salt
- 1 tbsp. extra-virgin olive oil

Directions:
1. Place asparagus bottoms in a large saucepan. Pour just the right amount of water. Make sure the asparagus are submerged vegetables.
2. Let boil. Once boiling, allow to simmer for a minute. Add in asparagus tops. Cook for 2 minutes more. Drain. Place inside the fridge until ready to use.
3. Meanwhile, put together palm sugar, light soy sauce, salt, and olive oil in a bowl. Mix until the sugar and salt dissolve.
4. Pour just the right amount of sauce all over chilled asparagus. Toss well to combine. Serve.

Squash Soup with Cashew Cheese

Ingredients:
- 1 Tbsp. olive oil
- 1 white onion, minced
- 1 garlic clove, minced
- 1 butternut squash, cubed
- 4 cups mushroom stock
- Pinch of kosher salt
- Pinch of white pepper, to taste

For garnish
- ¼ cup parsley, minced
- ¼ cup cashew cheese, divided

Directions:
1. Pour olive oil into a Dutch oven. Once the oil is hot, sauté white onion and garlic for 3 minutes or until limp and aromatic.
2. Add in butternut squash, mushroom stock, salt, and white pepper. Mix well. Bring to a boil.
3. Once boiling, reduce the heat and allow to simmer for 45 minutes. Turn off the heat.
4. Let cool for a few minutes before transferring to a food processor. Process until a smooth consistency is achieved. Adjust taste if needed.
5. To serve, ladle soup in bowls. Cool slightly before ladling into bowls. Garnish with parsley and cashew cheese on top.

Dinner Recipes

Hummus Bruschetta with Cucumber and Pomegranate

Ingredients:

- 2 slices wheat bread, lightly toasted
- 1½ Tbsp. hummus

For the toppings

- ½ Tbsp. tomato, diced
- ½ Tbsp. pomegranate seeds
- ½ Tbsp. cucumber, diced
- ¼ Tbsp. chives, minced
- Pinch of kosher salt
- Pinch of white pepper

Directions:

1. Spread hummus on the toasted bread. Place bruschetta in the oven toaster. Heat until warmed through.
2. Meanwhile, combine tomato, pomegranate seeds, cucumber, chives, salt, and white pepper in a mixing bowl.
3. Spread mixture on top of the bruschetta. Serve.

Scallops with Tomato-Leek Sauce

Ingredients:
- 2 tbsp. olive oil
- 2 garlic cloves, minced
- 1 cup snow peas, strings removed
- 2 leeks, white and light green parts
- 2 tomatoes, chopped
- 1 ½ cups scallops
- ¼ cup red wine
- 2 cups brown rice, cooked
- Pinch of salt
- Pinch of pepper

Directions:
1. Pour olive oil in a saucepan. Sauté garlic, snow peas, and leeks. Cook for 5 minutes.
2. Add in tomatoes, scallops, red wine, and brown rice. Allow mixture to simmer for 3 minutes. Season with salt and pepper. Mix until all ingredients are well-combined. Serve.

Grilled Catfish Fillets with Tomato Salad

Ingredients:

- ¼ lb. cherry tomatoes, quartered
- 2 salad tomatoes, ripe, cubed
- 2 green tomatoes, cubed
- 1 leek, minced
- Pinch, fresh cilantro, minced
- 1 tbsp. balsamic vinegar
- Pinch of salt
- Pinch of black pepper

- 4 catfish fillets
- 2 Tbsp. Spanish paprika powder
- ½ tsp. sea salt
- 1 tsp. red pepper flakes

Directions:
1. Set the grill pan on medium high heat.
2. Meanwhile, put together cherry tomatoes, green tomatoes, salad tomatoes, leek, cilantro, balsamic vinegar, salt, and pepper in a bowl. Toss until all ingredients are well-combined. Place inside the fridge until ready to serve.
3. In another bowl, mix Spanish paprika powder, salt, and red pepper flakes. Dredge catfish fillets on the marinade sauce.
4. Grill for 5 minutes on each side. Flip and grill for 3 minutes on the other side.
5. Transfer fish to a platter with aluminum foil. Allow to rest for 3 minutes.
6. To serve, place fish fillets on a platter with tomato salad on the side.

Baked Brussels Sprouts

Ingredients:

- 2 tbsp. olive oil, divided
- 1 lb brussels sprouts
- ½ onion, chopped finely
- ½ tsp. salt
- ½ tsp. ground black pepper

Directions:
1. Preheat the oven to 425 F. Lightly grease baking sheet with olive oil.
2. Place the steamer basket in a pot. Pour water. Bring to a boil.
3. Once boiling, put brussels in the steamer basket. Steam for 5 minutes.
4. Remove brussels from the pot. Drain and then transfer to a bowl.
5. Add in the remaining olive oil, onion, salt, and pepper.
6. Place inside the oven and bake for 15 minutes. Serve.

Stir-Fry Mixed Veggies

Ingredients:
- 3 tbsp.olive oil
- 1 package frozen mixed green vegetables
- 2 tbsp. water
- 2 tbsp. soy sauce
- 1 package fresh spinach

Directions:
1. Pour olive oil in a non-stick skillet. Add in frozen mixed greens. Stir fry for 5 minutes or until tender.
2. In the same skillet, pour water. Season with soy sauce. Allow to simmer for 3 minutes.
3. Stir in spinach. Steam for 3 minutes together with the mixed veggies, covered. Serve.

Spinach Salad with Mustard Dressing

Ingredients:

- 1/4 cup olive oil
- 1 butternut pumpkin, sliced
- 2 cups baby spinach leaves
- 3 red onions
- Pinch of salt
- Pinch of pepper
- 2 tbsp. apple cider vinegar
- 1 tbsp. wholegrain mustard
- 1 cup feta cheese

Directions:

1. Preheat the grill set over medium heat.
2. Baste pumpkin slices with olive oil, salt, and pepper. Grill until tender.
3. Transfer to a plate. Grill onion until translucent. Set aside.
4. Meanwhile, put together grilled pumpkin and onions in a bowl. Add in feta cheese and spinach.
5. For the dressing, mix wholegrain mustard, apple cider vinegar, and olive oil in a jar with tight-fitting lid. Shake well.
6. To serve, portion grilled veggies on plates. Drizzled in mustard dressing. Sprinkle feta cheese.

Simple Spinach and Kale Salad

Ingredients:

- 3 cups loosely packed spinach
- ½ cup kale leaves
- Dash of Worcestershire sauce
- 4 tsp. balsamic vinegar
- 1 ½ tsp. sugar
- 2 tsp. olive oil
- 1 oz. ~~Tofutti cheese~~ *mozerella cheese grated*

Directions:

1. Combine Worcestershire sauce, balsamic vinegar, sugar, and olive oil in a bowl. Mix well. Set aside.
2. Place kale and spinach in the bowl. Toss well to combine.
3. To serve, portion salads in plates. Pour dressing all over salad. Top with Tofutti cheese. Serve.

Tomato Salad Sandwich

Ingredients:

- 2 wheat bread, toasted
- 1 Tbsp. pesto sauce

For the Toppings

- 2 red cherry tomatoes, quartered
- 2 green cherry tomatoes, quartered
- Pinch of palm sugar, crumble
- ¼ tsp. balsamic vinegar
- ¼ tsp. apple cider vinegar
- Pinch of kosher salt
- Pinch of white pepper, to taste

Directions:

1. Spread pesto sauce on one side of the bread

2. Place inside the oven toaster and heat until warmed through.

3. Meanwhile, put together red cherry tomatoes, green cherry tomatoes, palm sugar, balsamic vinegar, and apple cider vinegar in a bowl.

4. Season with salt and pepper. Spread mixture on bread. Serve.

Broccoli Stem Noodles with Artichoke Pesto

Ingredients:
- 2 fresh broccoli stems, tender parts only
- Pinch of salt

Directions:
1. Scrape one side of broccoli stem using a vegetable peeler for the thick noodle. Turn broccoli a quarter-way to scrape that side, too.
2. Continue turning and scraping until stem is processed. Discard the rest.
3. Place vegetables in a colander. Sprinkle salt. Toss well to combine. Leave for 30 minutes to sweat.
4. Layer broccoli noodles on a towel. Roll tightly to remove salt and moisture. Do not rinse. Use as needed.

Artichoke Pesto Sauce

Ingredients:

- ½ cup canned, artichoke hearts
- ¼ cup cashew nuts, toasted
- 3 garlic cloves, minced
- 1 cup fresh basil leaves
- ¼ tsp. red pepper flakes
- 2 Tbsp. lemon juice, freshly squeezed
- ¾ cup extra virgin olive oil
- Pinch of kosher salt
- Pinch of white pepper, to taste

Directions:

1. Place artichoke hearts, cashew nuts, garlic cloves, basil leaves, red pepper flakes, lemon juice, olive oil, salt, and white pepper into the blender.
2. Process until smooth. Adjust taste if needed. Use with broccoli noodles.

Chicken with Vegetable Rice

Ingredients:
- 2 tbsp. olive oil
- 1 thumb-sized ginger, grated
- 1 garlic clove, minced
- 2 stalks leeks, minced, reserve some for garnish
- 2 lbs. chicken thigh fillets, diced
- 3 cups brown rice, cooked
- 1 head cauliflower, cut into bite-sized florets
- 1 can water chestnuts, quartered
- 1 red bell pepper, julienned
- ¾ cups chicken stock
- 1 tbsp. fish sauce
- Pinch of salt
- Pinch of black pepper
- ½ tbsp. cornstarch
- 4 tbsp. water
- 1 tsp. stevia

Directions:
1. Pour olive oil in a pan. Sauté ginger, garlic, and leeks for 3 minutes or until limp and fragrant. Set aside.
2. Add in chicken thigh fillets. Cook until golden brown. Place cauliflower, water chestnuts, red bell pepper, and chicken broth. Add in sautéed garlic, ginger, and leeks. Cook for 15 minutes, covered. Season mixture with fish sauce, salt, and pepper.
3. Meanwhile, dissolve cornstarch in water. Add in stevia. Bring mixture to a boil for 10 minutes.
4. To serve, place brown rice on a plate. Ladle chicken and veggies. Garnish with the remaining leeks. Serve.

Green Curry Chicken Pie

Ingredients:

- 1 tbsp. olive oil

- 1 tbsp. green curry paste

- 13 ½ oz. coconut milk

- 4 x ½ lb. chicken breast fillets, cut into ¾-inch pieces

- 1 ¾ lbs. butternut pumpkin, cut into 3/4-inch pieces

- 5 1/3 oz. baby spinach leaves

- 1 tbsp. fresh lime juice

- 1 tbsp. brown sugar

- 1 egg, lightly whisked

- 2 tsp. fish sauce

- 4 sheets pastry sheets

- Baby rocket leaves, for garnish

Directions:

1. Preheat the oven to 410 F.

2. Pour olive oil in a frying pan. Once hot, cook curry paste whilst stirring until aromatic. Add in coconut milk.

3. Bring it to a boil. Then, add the chicken breast and pumpkin pieces. Lower heat to medium and simmer while, occasionally stirring, for around 10 minutes or until pumpkin becomes fork tender.

4. Add spinach, fresh lime juice, brown sugar, and fish sauce into the mix. Stir the contents until spinach wilts.

5. Remove the pan from the heat and set aside to slightly cool down.

6. Transfer the chicken mixture into 4 rectangular pie tins (capacity of a cup each). Brush tin edges with the beaten egg.

7. Fold each pastry sheet in half. Brush each side of the pastry sheet. Top each pie tin with a sheet. Cut pastry sheets 2 slits on top of the pie. Brush the tops with the beaten egg.

8. Bake for 20 minutes or until the pastry becomes golden and puffed. Remove it from the oven and serve with baby rocket leaves.

Almond-crusted Red Snapper

Ingredients:

- 8 red snapper fillets

- 2 eggs, beaten

- 1 cup ground almonds

- 2 cups Parmesan, grated

- 1 tsp. lemon pepper

- 1 tsp. garlic salt

- 1/4 cup all-purpose flour

- 6 tbsp. butter

- 8 sprigs parsley

- 8 fresh lemon wedges

- Pinch of salt

Instructions

1. Combine garlic salt, beaten eggs, and lemon pepper until blended.

2. In a shallow dish, put together the ground almonds and a cup of parmesan cheese.

3. Dust the fillets with flour. Shake off any excess.

4. Dip the dusted fillets in the egg mixture. Press it into the almond mixture.

5. In a large frying pan, melt the butter over medium-high heat. Fry the fillets in it for 2 minutes each side or until golden brown.

6. Lower the heat to medium. If desired, season the fillets with salt. Sprinkle the cooked fillets with the remaining Parmesan. Cover the frying pan for around 5 minutes to melt the cheese.

7. Transfer the fillets on a serving dish. Garnish with parsley and lemon wedges. Serve.

Grilled Chicken Breast

Ingredients:

- Olive oil, for cooking

- ½ bunch rainbow chard

- 3 chicken breast

- 1 lemon, halved

- Pinch of salt

- Pinch of pepper, to taste

Directions:

1. Pour olive oil in a wok. Once hot, sauté the rainbow chard. Season with salt and pepper for 3 minutes or until wilted.

2. Squeeze in a bit of lemon juice. Set aside.

3. Pat chicken meat with paper towels to dry. Season with salt and pepper to taste. Grill on a well-oiled grill until desired doneness is achieved.

4. Let meat rest for half the time it was grilled. Slice and sprinkle with a pinch of salt. Serve with the rainbow chard on the side.

Meat Pies

Ingredients:

- 1 1/5 lbs. ground chicken

- 1 medium onion, chopped

- 1 cup of water, divided

- 3 cups chicken stock

- ¼ cup ketchup

- 2 tsp. Worcestershire sauce

- Pepper to taste

- ½ tsp. oregano

- 1 pinch of ground nutmeg

- 3 tbsp. all-purpose flour

- 2 sheets of puff pastry

- 1 egg, beaten

Directions:

1. Preheat the oven to 425 F.

2. In a frying pan over medium-high heat, brown the ground chicken and onion.

3. Add ¾ cup of water, chicken stock, ketchup, pepper, oregano, ground nutmeg, and Worcestershire sauce. Let it boil.

4. Once it boils, cover the pan for 15 minutes.

5. Mix the remaining water with the flour. Blend until it gets a smooth texture. Add it to the mix in the frying pan. Stir the contents and remove from heat. Let it cool.

6. Grease a pie dish and line it with the puff pastry sheets. Add the cooled mixture as filling. Brush the edges of the pastry with the beaten egg. Cover

the top with more pastry sheets. Seal the edges by pressing it down with a fork.

7. Trim excess pastry and brush the top with the remaining beaten egg.

8. Put it in the oven and bake for 15 minutes. Then, reduce heat to 350 F and bake for 25 minutes or until pastry becomes golden brown.

9. Serve with vegetables, salad, or mashed potatoes.

Chicken Parmigiana

Ingredients:

- 2 chicken breast fillet,skinless,halved

- 16 oz. spaghetti sauce

- 1 egg, beaten

- 2 oz. dry breadcrumbs

- 2 oz. mozzarella cheese, shredded

- ¼ cup Parmesan, grated

Directions:

1. Preheat the oven to 350 F. Lightly grease a baking sheet.

2. Place beaten egg in a bowl. Put breadcrumbs in another bowl.

3. Dip chicken in the egg and then the breadcrumbs. Place coated chicken breast fillets on the baking sheet.

4. Place inside the oven and bake for 40 minutes. Pour half of the sauce over the baking dish.

5. Put cooked chicken over the spaghetti sauce. Mix well. Cover with mozzarella and Parmesan cheese. Place back in the oven and bake for another 20 minutes. Serve.

Oatmeal-Crusted Vegetables and Chicken Wings (serve this every once in a while)

Ingredients:
- 1 cup almond flour, finely milled
- 2 eggs, lightly beaten
- 1 cup steel-cut oats
- Olive oil, for frying
- 4 chicken wings
- 1 sweet potato, sliced into slivers
- 1 carrot, sliced into long slivers
- 1 aubergine, sliced into slivers
- 6 green beans, sliced into slivers
- 1 tsp. Spanish paprika
- 1 tsp. salt
- 1 tsp. ground black pepper

Directions:
1. Season chicken wings, sweet potato, carrots aubergine, and green beans, with paprika, salt, and pepper. Set aside for 20 minutes.
2. Meanwhile, pour almond flour, eggs, and oats in separate bowls. Dip vegetables and chicken wings in this order: almond flour first, then eggs, and then oats.
3. Pour olive oil in a pan. Fry vegetables and chicken wings until golden brown. Drain on paper towels. Serve.

Papaya, Grapes, and Pineapple Salad

Ingredients:
- 2 cups ripe papaya, cubed
- 2 red grapes, halved
- 2 green grapes, halved
- 1 can pineapple, do not drain
- 1 tsp. palm sugar, crumbled
- Pinch of salt

Directions:
1. Put together papaya, red and green grapes, pineapple tidbits with juices in a salad bowl.
2. Toss well to combine. Place inside the fridge for 30 minutes to 1 hour.
3. To serve, spoon equal portions in salad bowls. Sprinkle salt and palm sugar on top. Serve.

Mandarin Oranges Salad with Soy Vinaigrette
Ingredients:
- ¼ cup walnuts, chopped

For the vinaigrette
- 1 tsp. garlic, grated
- 1 tsp. ginger, grated
- 3 tbsp. light soy sauce
- ½ cup apple cider vinegar
- 1 tbsp. honey
- 1½ tsp. chilli oil
- 2 tbsp. extra virgin olive oil
- 1 tsp. sesame oil
- Pinch of salt
- Pinch of pepper

For the salad
- 2 cups red cabbage, julienned
- 6 cups napa cabbage, julienned
- 1 cup carrot, julienned
- ½ cup leeks, minced
- ½ cup water chestnuts, sliced
- 1 can Mandarin oranges, drained
- ½ cup walnuts, chopped

Directions:
1. Put together garlic, ginger, soy sauce, apple cider vinegar, honey, chilli oil, olive oil, sesame oil, salt, and pepper in a bowl. Whisk. Set aside.
2. In another bowl, combine red cabbage, carrot, napa cabbage, leeks, water chestnuts, and Mandarin oranges. Drizzle in just the right amount of vinaigrette. Toss well to combine.
3. To serve, place equal amounts in salad plates. Drizzle in the remaining vinaigrette. Sprinkle with walnuts on top.

Thyme and Lemon Sweet Potato Soup

Ingredients:
- 2 tbsp. thyme
- Lemon juice
- 1 tbsp. coconut oil
- 4 bell peppers, diced
- 2 cups sweet potato, mashed
- 1 onion, diced
- 4 cups vegetable broth
- 1 tsp. cumin
- Pinch of salt
- Pinch of pepper

Directions:
1. Pour coconut oil in a saucepan. Sauté onions and bell peppers for 3 minutes or until tender.
2. Meanwhile, combine sweet potato, half of the vegetable stock, peppers, and cumin in a food processor. Process until smooth.
3. Transfer mixture to the saucepan. Let it simmer for 20 minutes. Add in thyme and lemon juice. Season with salt and pepper. Serve.

Fish Stew with Tomatoes

Ingredients:
- 1 ½ lbs halibut fish
- 1 can diced tomatoes with juice
- 1 tbsp. extra-virgin olive oil
- 2 onions, chopped finely
- 3 garlic cloves, minced
- 1 fennel bulb, diced
- 2 cups fish stock
- ½ cup black olives, chopped
- 2 tsp. dried Italian seasoning
- 1 tsp. sea salt
- 1 tsp. peppercorns
- 1 jalapeño pepper, diced

Directions:
1. Pour olive oil in a pan. Sauté garlic and onions for 3 minutes or until limp and aromatic. Stir in fennel. Season with salt, pepper, and Italian seasoning. Sauté for 3 minutes.
2. Pour diced tomatoes with juice and fish stock. Cover and cook for 1 hour.
3. Add in halibut fish, jalapeno pepper, and olives. Cook for another 15 minutes.
4. To serve, ladle stew in soup bowls. Serve.

Salmon and Barley Soup

Ingredients:
- 12 oz. salmon fillet
- 1 tbsp. olive oil
- ¾ cup barley, quick-cooking
- 1 cup onions, chopped
- 1 cup canned tomatoes with juice
- 1 cup green beans
- 4 cups vegetable broth
- 1 cup carrots, chopped
- 2 cups water
- ¼ tsp. salt
- Pinch of ground black pepper

Directions:
1. Pour olive oil in a large saucepan. Sauté onions, carrots, and green beans for 5 minutes or until tender and translucent.
2. Pour water, tomatoes with juice, vegetable broth, barley, and salt. Allow to simmer for 5 minutes or until tender.
3. Stir in salmon fillets. Cook for 5 minutes. Season with salt and pepper. Adjust seasoning if needed. Serve.

Asparagus Rice

Ingredients:
- 3 cups brown rice, cooked
- 2 cups vegetable stock
- ½ lb thick-stemmed asparagus
- ¼ cup fresh parsley, minced, for garnish
- Pinch of salt
- Pinch of black pepper

Directions:
1. Pour brown rice and asparagus in a rice cooker. Season with salt and pepper. Pour vegetable stock. Secure the lid. Press the "cook" function on the rice cooker.
2. Wait until the machine automatically shifts to warm. Turn off the machine.
3. To serve, ladle just the right portions in bowls. Garnish with fresh parsley on top.

Baked Salmon with Kale Chips

Ingredients:
- 1 lb. fresh kale leaves
- 2 salmon fillets
- Spanish paprika
- Pinch of salt
- Pinch of pepper
- 2 tbsp. olive oil
- ¼ cup Parmesan cheese, grated
- ½ lemon juice, freshly squeezed

Directions
1. For the kale chips, preheat the oven to 350 degrees F.
2. Season kale with salt and drizzle in just the right amount of olive oil. Layer kale leaves on a baking sheet. Place inside the oven and bake for 10 minutes.
3. Remove from the oven and let cool for 5 minutes.
4. To cook the salmon fillets, place on a baking dish. Season with paprika, salt, and pepper. Bake for 20 minutes.
5. Remove from the oven and cover with aluminium foil to rest for 5 minutes.
6. To serve, place salmon fillet on a plate. Squeeze in lemon juice. Place kale chips on the side.

Sweet and Sour Chicken Fillets

Ingredients:
- 8 chicken breast fillets, cubed
- 1 tbsp. onion powder
- 1 tbsp. garlic powder
- 1 tbsp. Spanish paprika
- Pinch of salt
- Pinch of white pepper
- 2 cups almond flour, finely milled
- ¼ cup self-rising flour
- ⅛ tsp. baking powder
- 1 egg, whisked
- ¼ cup cornstarch
- 1 cup cold water
- 2 tsp. coconut oil, divided
- 2 onions, quartered
- 2 garlic cloves, minced
- 1 red bell pepper, cubed
- 1 green bell pepper, cubed
- Pinch of sea salt

For the Sauce
- 1 can pineapple tidbits
- 2 tbsp. sugar, crumbled
- 1 carrot, sliced into flowers
- ½ cup rice wine vinegar
- 1 tsp. cornstarch
- 1 cup water
- Pinch of sea salt
- Pinch of white pepper

Directions:
1. Combine garlic powder, onion powder, Spanish paprika, salt and pepper in a zip lock bag.
2. Put chicken fillets inside the bag and massage. Make sure all fillets are evenly coated. Place inside the fridge for 1 hour or overnight for the flavors to meld.

3. Meanwhile, put together baking powder, almond flour, egg, self-rising flour, cornstarch, and water in a bowl. Mix well. Place chicken until well coated.
4. Pour coconut oil in a pan. Slide breaded chicken and cook for 3 minutes or until golden brown. Drain on paper towels. Set aside.
5. In the same pan, pour remaining coconut oil. Sauté garlic and onion for 3 minutes or until limp. Add in red and green bell peppers. Season with salt. Stir in cooked chicken fillet. Cook for 1 minute. Remove from heat.
6. Combine water and cornstarch in a small bowl. Add in pineapple tidbits, sugar, carrots, rice wine vinegar, salt, and pepper. Pour mixture over the saucepan.
7. Cook for 3 minutes or until the sauce thickens. Pour sauce over chicken. Serve.

Chicken Salad with Soy Vinegar Vinaigrette

Ingredients:

For the Vinaigrette
- 1 tsp. soy sauce
- ¼ cup rice wine vinegar
- ¼ tbsp. palm sugar
- 1 garlic clove, grated
- 1 tsp. ginger, grated
- 1 tbsp. sesame oil

For the Salad
- ½ cup red cabbage, julienned
- 1 leek, minced
- 2 cups roasted chicken, diced
- ¼ cup carrots, grated
- 2 heads Romaine lettuce, torn into pieces
- ¼ cup edamame, cooked
- Pinch of sea salt
- Pinch of white pepper
- ¼ cup almond slivers, toasted

Directions:
1. Put together soy sauce, rice wine vinegar, garlic clove, ginger, palm sugar, and sesame oil in a bowl. Stir mixture well.
2. Meanwhile, mix Romaine lettuce, red cabbage, edamame, roasted chicken, carrots, leek, and almond slivers. Season with salt and pepper.
3. To serve, portion salad in plates. Drizzle in just the right amount of vinaigrette. Serve.

Desserts and Snacks

Chia Seed and Apple Jam Parfait

Ingredients:
- 1 tbsp. cashew nuts, chopped

For the Parfait base
- 2 tbsp. chia seeds
- 1 overripe banana, mashed
- ⅛ tsp. nutmeg powder
- ½ tsp. cinnamon powder
- 1¼ cups almond milk, chilled

For the Apple jam
- 2 apples, diced
- ¾ cup organic apple juice, unsweetened
- ⅛ tsp. nutmeg powder
- ¾ tsp. cinnamon powder
- 2 tbsp. chia seeds
- Pinch of salt

Directions:
1. Combine chia seeds, banana, nutmeg powder, cinnamon powder, and almond milk in a bowl. Place inside the fridge to chill until ready to use.
2. For the apple jam, prepare a large saucepan. Place apples, apple juice, nutmeg powder, cinnamon powder, chia seeds, and salt. Bring to a boil.
3. Once boiling, reduce the heat and allow to simmer for 20 minutes. Turn off the heat.
4. Mash half of the jam using a potato masher. Let cool.

Apricots and Apples Puddings

Ingredients:
- 1 cup dates
- 1 cup apricots
- 1 apple, chopped
- 1 cup dried cherries
- ½ tsp. ground nutmeg
- 1 orange, zest and juice
- 2 tbsp. brown sugar
- ½ cup olive oil
- 1/2 cup applesauce
- 75g self-rising flour
- 2 cups ground almonds
- 75g breadcrumbs
- 2 tbsp. almond milk
- 1 tsp. vanilla extract

Directions:
1. Preheat the oven to 300 F. Lightly grease muffin tins.
2. Mix dates, apricots, apple, cherries, nutmeg, orange juice and zest in a saucepan. Bring to a boil for 3 minutes. Set aside.
3. In another bowl, put together brown sugar and olive oil. Stir well. Add in applesauce, flour, ground almonds, breadcrumbs, almond milk, and vanilla extract. Mix until all ingredients come together.
4. Put equal amounts in muffin tins. Bake for 1 hour or until the pudding is firm. Let cool before serving.

Watermelon Lollies

Ingredients:

- ½ cup watermelon, cubed
- 2 tbsp. lemon juice, freshly squeezed
- ½ cup water
- 1 tbsp. stevia

Directions:
1. Place watermelon cubes in a blender. Process until smooth. Divide equal amounts into ice pop containers.
2. Place inside the freezer for 1 hour.
3. Meanwhile, mix water, lemon juice, and stevia in a small bowl. Mix. Pour over frozen watermelon lollies. Put pop sticks. Freeze for another 1-2 hours.
4. Pry out lollies and then serve.

Coconut Bread Twist

Ingredients:

- 2 cups coconut flour, finely-milled
- ½ cup chilled coconut butter
- ½ cup coconut flakes
- 2 egg, whisked
- 1 drop vanilla extract
- 1 Tbsp. heaping all-purpose flour
- Olive oil
- cold water, only if needed

Toppings

- 2 Tbsp. palm sugar, crumbled
-
- ¼ cup coconut meat, grated

Directions:

1. Process butter into coconut flour until it resembles breadcrumbs. Add in coconut flakes, all-purpose flour, eggs, and vanilla extract. Mix until the dough comes together.
2. Pour olive oil in a pan. Once hot, slide in a few breadsticks at a time and cook until golden brown. Drain on paper towels.
3. Serve with crumbled palm sugar, and coconut meat.

Cherry Ripe Bites

Ingredients:

- ½ cup fresh cherries, halved, pitted
- ¾ cup desiccated coconut
- 2 tbsp. dry-roasted strawberry powder
- 1 tbsp. melted coconut oil
- ¼ cup dark chocolate, melted

Directions:

1. Preheat oven to 325 F.
2. Spread cherries with cut-side up on a baking sheet lined with parchment paper. Roast in the oven for 20 minutes.
3. Blend roasted cherries and dry-roasted powder together until smooth.
4. Add desiccated coconut and coconut oil into the blender. Blend to combine.
5. Pour the blended mixture into a silicone ice cube tray. Refrigerate for an hour to set.
6. Once set, remove the set mixture from the mold.
7. Dip the cherry ripe bites into the melted dark chocolate. Then, lay it on parchment paper to set.
8. Store in an airtight container and refrigerate for storage.

Blueberry Lemon Muffins

Ingredients:

For the Dry ingredients
- 1½ tsp. baking soda
- 2 cups all-purpose flour, unbleached
- 2 tsp. lemon zest
- ½ tsp. salt

For the Wet ingredients
- ⅓ cup coconut oil
- 1 cup rice milk
- ¾ cup palm sugar, crumbled
- 1 tbsp. lemon juice, freshly squeezed

- 1½ cup blueberries, rinsed, drained well

Directions:
1. Preheat the oven to 375°F. Line paper liners in muffin tins.
2. Combine baking soda, all-purpose flour, lemon zest, and salt in a bowl.
3. Place coconut oil, rice milk, palm sugar, and lemon juice in another bowl. Stir well.
4. Fold in blueberries. Spoon equal portions into 11 muffin tins. Bake for 25 minutes. Remove from the oven.
5. Cool muffins on cake rack before serving.

Apricot Balsamic Jam

Ingredients:
- 2 lbs. apricots, diced
- 3 tbsp. balsamic vinegar
- ½ lemon, freshly juiced
- 1 cup maple syrup
- ¼ cup water

Directions:
1. Place apricots, balsamic vinegar, lemon, maple syrup, and water in a large saucepan. Allow mixture to boil.
2. Once boiling, reduce the heat and allow to simmer for 10 minutes.
3. Mash fruits using a spoon. Stir frequently. Cook until most of the liquid has evaporated. Turn off the heat.
4. Allow to cool at room temperature before storing in airtight container. Serve as needed.

Almond Jelly Fruit Salad

Ingredients:
- coconut oil, for greasing
- 2 pouches unflavoured gelatine
- 2 cups almond milk, unsweetened
- 2 tsp. palm sugar, crumbled
- 2 cups water
- ½ tsp. almond extract

Fruit salad
- 1 pear, diced
- 2 cherries, halved
- 1 apple, diced
- 1 banana, sliced into thick medallions
- ¼ cup almond slivers, toasted

Directions:
1. Lightly grease a baking dish with coconut oil. Combine unflavored gelatin, palm sugar, almond milk, and water in saucepan. Stir until the gelatin dissolves.
2. Allow the mixture to simmer while stirring. Gelatin is done when it sticks to the back of the spoon. Turn off the heat.
3. Add in almond extract. Pour gelatin into the baking dish. Let cool for a few minutes. Seal with saran wrap. Place inside the fridge to chill before slicing into cubes.
4. To serve, combine apples, cherries, banana, and pear in a salad bowl. Garnish with toasted almonds on top.

Soy Berries Parfait

Ingredients:
- 2 cups soy milk
- ½ pack graham crackers
- ½ tsp. ground cinnamon
- 1 cup blueberries
- 1 cup strawberries, halved

Directions:

1. Place graham crackers and cinnamon into the food processor. Process until crumbly.
2. To assemble, pour graham cracker crumbs to serve as parfait's base. Pour soy milk. Dot with strawberries, blueberries, and graham crackers. Finish with some crumbs of graham crackers.
3. Place inside the fridge to cool for 2 hours or until ready to serve.

Cranberry Flax Balls

Ingredients:
- 1 tbsp. ground flax seed
- 1 tbsp. chia seeds
- 1 cup date
- 1/2 cup honey
- Pinch of salt
- 1 1/2 cups oats
- 1 cup pistachio nuts, shelled
- 1 cup dried cranberries
- 1/3 cup white chocolate chips

Directions:
1. Line a baking pan with parchment paper.
2. Meanwhile, combine dates, chia seeds, ground flax seeds, honey, and salt in a food processor. Pulse until well-combined.
3. Transfer mixture to a bowl. Add in dried cranberries, oats, pistachios, and white chocolate chips. Place inside the fridge for at 30 minutes.
4. Once cooled, shape into balls. Arrange on the baking pan. Allow to cool for 30 minutes before cutting. Place inside the fridge until ready to serve.

Fresh Avocado Salad

Ingredients:
- 2 ripe avocado, cubed
- ½ cup stevia
- 1 cup almond milk

Directions:
1. In a mixing bowl, combine avocado, stevia, and almond milk. Stir well.
2. Chill for 1 hour or until ready to use.
3. To serve, place equal portions in bowls.

Food and Exercise Diary

Day 1

Breakfast
Lunch / Including afternoon snack
Dinner
Exercise
How do you feel?

Measure Yourself

Starting weight: _____ lbs.

Starting waistline: _____ inches

Day 2

Breakfast
Lunch / Including afternoon snack
Dinner
Exercise
How do you feel?

Day 3

Breakfast
Lunch / Including afternoon snack
Dinner
Exercise
How do you feel?

Day 4

Breakfast
Lunch / Including afternoon snack
Dinner
Exercise
How do you feel?

Day 5

Breakfast
Lunch / Including afternoon snack
Dinner
Exercise
How do you feel?

Day 6

Breakfast
Lunch / Including afternoon snack
Dinner
Exercise
How do you feel?

Day 7

Breakfast
Lunch / Including afternoon snack
Dinner
Exercise
How do you feel?

Measure Yourself

Weight after 1 week: _____ lbs.

Waistline after 1 week: _____ inches

Week 2

Day 8

Breakfast
Lunch / Including afternoon snack
Dinner
Exercise
How do you feel?

Day 9

Breakfast
Lunch / Including afternoon snack
Dinner
Exercise
How do you feel?

Day 10

Breakfast
Lunch / Including afternoon snack
Dinner
Exercise
How do you feel?

Day 11

Breakfast
Lunch / Including afternoon snack
Dinner
Exercise
How do you feel?

Day 12

Breakfast
Lunch / Including afternoon snack
Dinner
Exercise
How do you feel?

Day 13

Breakfast
Lunch / Including afternoon snack
Dinner
Exercise
How do you feel?

Day 14

Breakfast
Lunch / Including afternoon snack
Dinner
Exercise
How do you feel?

Measure Yourself

Weight after 2 weeks: _____ lbs.

Waistline after 2 weeks: _____ inches

"Up your game. You can sign up for a race. It doesn't matter if you're slow or fast, or you come in last. The idea is to set a goal for yourself. Make a commitment and stick to it."